A New Healthy Food Plan

Elizabeth Carrell

IN MEMORY OF

RODNEY CARRELL

DIED AT THE AGE OF 49 FROM DIABETES

A NEW HEALTHY FOOD PLAN

(For the whole family)

1 INTRODUCTION

Good exercise and nutrition *is* the best solution for a long and healthy life. Some of the questions to be considered are: Is low-carb diet a good diet to use? Can white bread and sugar be a good source from the five-food group? How does one start in an exercise routine? Herbal supplements, are they harmful or not?

Low-carb diet means a high fat diet. Warner (2004) stated, "That means a blue cheese-topped steak, one of the offerings on T.G.I. Friday's Atkins-Approved menu, is still going to pack more fat and calories than a grilled chicken from the regular menu (para 12)." So, what should people order at restaurants? Meat or chicken that is grilled will get most of the fat off (grease), baked potatoes, and grilled, boiled, or fresh vegetables are the best foods to order at restaurants. Here is what Halton (2007) stated,

"One possible explanation why diets that replaced carbs with animal protein and fat were not associated with

higher heart-disease risk is that the adverse effects of animal products might be counter-balanced by reducing refined carbohydrates and; the quality of fat and carbohydrate is more important than quantity" (para 7).

Some people do not know how to eat a low-carb diet without high fat. One of the best way to help lose weight is by eating a low-carb diet by eating good healthy meals with little sugar, candies, and sodas and stay away from margarine, corn oil, shortening, safflower oil, soybean oil, and cottonseed oil and eat moderately. The five food groups that are needed to stay healthy are protein, low-fat oils, fruits and vegetables, whole grains, and dairy food.

2 THE MEAT GROUP

Protein consists of lean beef, eggs, pork, fish, skinless chicken ,nuts, turkey, and beans. A person needs to eat three to four servings of fish and beans a week. Eat four to six tablespoons of peanut butter, five days a week and be guilt-free by losing weight. Unsalted peanuts and peanut butter are a good source of protein.

Which of the meats have vitamins, calcium, and zinc? Pork has Thiamin. On the other hand, beef, salmon, and turkey has Riboflavin. Oysters, shrimp, and lobster have Iodine in them. Which fish has calcium? It is Sardines. Other fish that have Vitamin B12 are mussels, crabs, clams, and swordfish. Lentils and cashews have Pantothenic acid. Believe it or not, almonds have calcium. Legumes, eggs, and peanut butter have biotin.

Walnuts lowers breast cancer, sunflower seeds lowers cholesterol, peanuts helps control diabetes and reduces cholesterol. In fact, most nuts do reduce cholesterol. Did anyone know that pistachios help reduce lung cancer?

3 FRUITS AND VEGETABLES

Adding green vegetables like broccoli, green beans, salad, spinach, and collard green to complement a meal with pasta will curb down the carbs. There are exceptional cookbooks to use and recipes to help curb down the carbs. Some people are tired and have no energy! In order to function properly, a good workout and eat the food that has magnesium. Such food to eat is halibut and shellfish, black beans, whole grains, avocados, nuts, and spinach.

Green tea and blueberries slows aging and prevents cancer. Blueberries have Vitamin C and E and more antioxidant than any other fresh fruits and vegetables. The people who are over 65 years old that ate the blueberries have better motor skills than those who did not. Have a bowl of fruits on the table plus; fix up a tray of raw vegetables with a low-fat cheese dip and set it on the counter for the family to snack on. For an exceptional home remedy for a scratchy throat is eating fresh pineapple. The best time to eat the pineapple is to eat it early and eat, three ½ cups each day for a day or two.

It is not enough to eat just fruits and vegetables! After eating fruits and vegetables, it will take several hours for a person to get all the nutrients that is needed for the body. Juice Therapy is freshly squeezed fruits and vegetables is an excellent source of nutrients for the body which goes into the bloodstream is very digestible and better than taking multiple vitamins been used for many years by naturopaths and treats any kind of ailments. Celery juice is good for vascular system and can include with other vegetables by drinking eight-ounces of juice, two times a day. Make an exceptional fruit smoothie drink! The commercial drinks that are in tins, cartons, and bottles are not as good as they lose their nutrients. Pomegranate juice is an exceptional juice to drink, as it is high in antioxidant along with Vitamin A, C, E, and folic acid and; helps reduce cholesterol, any types of cancer, improve the blood flow, and works well as a blood thinner. Before drinking pomegranate juice, check with the doctor first. Cranberry juice is an exceptional juice to drink, as it is high in Vitamin C and fiber. To get the best results in cranberry juice is to sweeten with apple juice. This makes an exceptional combination of juices and very tasty and; is an exceptional protection from flu, colds, and will reduce infections. Now, strawberries are high in fiber with antioxidants, Vitamin A, C, B6, and B12, protein, calcium, magnesium, folic acid, and high in potassium. Make an exceptional tasty juice by combining blueberries, strawberries, and raspberries together. Internal Health Library (2006) stated that lime juice was used for scurvy in the sixteenth century and saved thousands of sailors' lives on their long voyages around the world.

Vegetables are loaded with Vitamins and minerals. Broccoli, spinach, carrots, sweet potatoes, butternut squash, and pumpkins all have Vitamin A. The vegetables that have Vitamin K are broccoli, carrots, and spinach. For the next set of vegetables that have Vitamin E are broccoli and spinach. In addition, lima beans, cauliflower, green peppers and potatoes have Vitamin B6. Brussels sprouts, green beans, turnip greens, and broccoli have calcium.

Now, there are some fruit that have Vitamin A. They are cantaloupe, mangoes, and apricots. The fruits that have Vitamin E are mangoes, blackberries, and apples. Which one has potassium? They are bananas, avocados, dried fruits, and tomatoes.

4 WHOLE GRAINS

Some people do not know that eating white bread is not good for the body because; it loses its immune system, have constipation, and high risk of cancer. What kind of grain should people eat? Use high-fiber whole grain breakfast, barley, oatmeal, and raisin bran, whole wheat bread, chickpeas, plain popcorn, sweet potatoes, an apple, strawberries, and yogurt to add for an exceptional diet plan. Cook brown rice ahead and freeze for other meals.

5 FATS, OIL, SWEETS, AND MILK GROUP

The best kinds of oil are low-fat oils that consist of olive oil, canola oil, peanut oil, one gram of saturated fat per tablespoon, Tran's fat-free margarine, and olive oil sprayer.

Milk is not harmful when it comes to three a day. People who choose 1% milk will get the benefit of calcium each day. Three a day can be a combination of cheese, milk, and yogurt. The other combinations are mashed potatoes, creamed soups, and instant hot chocolate. To get double calcium is evaporated milk that can be used to make creamed chowders. Raw milk is not good to drink as it may cause disease and death. To stay hydrated is to drink eight 8-ounces of glasses of water a day, a combination of tea, juice, and milk. Milk and cheese have calcium. In fact, milk also has Vitamin D.

White sugar is not good for the body! Some people do not know that white sugar is not good as; it is refined.

"Refined sugar is an extremely high glycemic food; it hits your bloodstream hard and can have severe impact on blood sugar, insulin levels, digestive enzyme count, weight, and the pancreas". Stated Anisman-Reiner (2006, para 3). Brown sugar consists of white sugar and molasses. What kind of sugar should people us for cooking? Instead of using white sugar, substitute it with maple syrup or honey. Raw honey is good for soothing sore throat, kills bacteria, and upset stomach. Anisman-Reiner (2006) stated that there are traces of zinc and manganese which is good for the heart and cholesterol and; the best grade to use is Grade C (para 4)".

Eat honey and cinnamon to avoid heart disease. Instead of eating jelly and jam on bread, mix honey cinnamon and spread on bread or toast. Cinnamon and honey cures most diseases. Some of them are arthritis, bladder infections, cholesterol, hearing loss, pimples, indigestion, weight loss, and colds. Cinnamon can be used for boosting memory, treat toothaches; eliminate bad breath, headaches, and migraine pain.

Apple cider vinegar is a cure-all? Drink a glass of water mixed with vinegar, molasses, and honey each to get a full head of hair. Vinegar will help a person lose weight. Vinegar fights off illness? Use apple cider vinegar for arthritis.

Use Flax seed oil vinegar for arthritis! Other benefits for flax seed oil are skin problems, diabetes, lowering cholesterol levels, improve immune system, fight obesity, and treat dandruff. Raw onions are good for insect stings. Use aloe Vera for burn pain. Clove oil can be used for toothache pain.

.

6 SUPPLEMENTS AND HERBS

Herbal supplements may be harmful! Herbal supplement is good to take but when taking multiple herbal supplements; it may cause flu like system, lack of sleep, liver and kidney, or heart problems. Single herbal supplement are an exceptional way to use versus multiple supplements. One of the herbal supplements is good for migraine headache is Feverfew. To get the best results in taking Feverfew, one must start taking it every day. Cleveland Clinic (2002) stated, "Although herbs seem harmless, they can be potentially dangerous, especially to anyone taking medication for a heart problem (para 2)." Before taking any herbal supplements ask the doctor and; let the pharmacist know.

Harvard Health Publications (2005) stated,

"Clinical guidelines suggest that if an individual has not lost at least a pound a week in the first month on a weight-loss medication, she's unlikely to benefit from the drug (para, 15, p 1)."

Here are some supplements that may be helpful. Vitamin B complex aids in the nervous and digestive system, and helps the skin, nails, and hair stay in good condition. Glucosamine Sulphate is highly effective to aid in arthritis pain, joint stress, and speed healing of sports injuries.

7 READ LABELS AND GENERAL HEALTH

While reading labels, keep in mind what to watch out for. What does a person's doctor want him or her to watch for in labels? Is it cholesterol, fats, and sugar? What about sodium? Which cereal is high in fiber?

Internal Health Library (2006) stated, "Indeed, a report by the British Ministry of Health & Public Service Laboratory back in the 1950's stated that:

'Juices are valuable in relief of hypertension, cardiovascular and kidney diseases and obesity. Good results have been obtained with large amounts, up to one litre daily, in the treatment of petic ulceration also in the treatment of chronic diarrhea, colitis, and toxemia of gastro and intestinal origin… The high buffering capacities of the juices reveal that they are very valuable in the treatment of hyperchlrohydria (excessive production of hydrochloric acid in the stomach). Milk has often been used for this purpose, but spinach juice, juices of cabbage, kale and parsley were found to be superior to milk for this purpose.' (para6)."

Reduce the risk of Alzheimer's disease! Taking a higher dose of Vitamin C and E will lower the chance of getting Alzheimer's. Additionally, doing exercising, reading, and staying healthy will help to keep the mind at work. Here are more ways to avoid Alzheimer's disease. One of the fun things to do is go to an art gallery or do some art work. Dancing or learn how to play a new instrument. Doing puzzles or crossword puzzle is fun to do. The main thing is stay positive, learn a new skill, and above all, have a social life. Stay sharp! There are two more things for a person to stay sharp. First, drink apple juice and last, protect your head. A blow to the head, even a mild one may increase odds of dementia years later. Eat fiber-rich cereal and cheese to prevent Alzheimer's.

Honey for colds! Take 2 ounces of honey a day for two days to help reduce the length of cold. How does one take care of a sore throat? Drink warm tea with honey and lemon. Build immune system up! How? Eat 2 6 ounce of yogurt and 2 glasses of orange juice a day.

How does one get any sleep? Use lavender or jasmine fragrance for a good night's sleep. Foods that fight stress! They are dark chocolate, warm skim milk, oatmeal, salmon, walnuts, sunflower seeds, spinach, and blueberries. Take a break, exercise, and meditate. Work out for thirty minutes before bed! Didn't get enough sleep on work days. Then, take extra hours of sleep on days off. Using a nightlight will help with insomnia, too. Take a shoulder massage for ten minutes, release tight muscles, and solve insomnia.

Foods that reduce colon cancer! Eat broccoli, Brussels sprouts, kale, and cabbage. Add whole grains by eating a high fiber diet. How to protect oneself from cancer! Here are the four ways: balance nutrition, watch your waist, don't smoke, and skip alcohol. In addition, other ways to protect for getting cancer are plenty of sleep, exercise, smile, drink pomegranate juice, eat beans, lentils, berries, artichokes, prunes, gala, red delicious and granny smith apples, black plums, and russet potatoes.

People who are diabetic have to make some changes in his or her life. This means no sodas, lose weight, exercise, and eat high fiber and whole grains, and no smoking.

How does one relieve joint pain? Here are a few ways to reduce joint pain. First of all, exercise, second don't push body past its limits, and last lose weight by getting on a high fiber and low fat diet. High fiber means eat lots of vegetables and some fruits with a small portion of meat.

Ways to improve an underactive thyroid! Eat Brussels sprouts, kale, broccoli, and cauliflower, 1-cup serving three times a week. Three supplements to take are Vitamin B2, Vitamin B3, and Vitamin B 6. These three vitamins will help boost a person's energy.

How does one get rid of varicose veins? Here are five ways to eliminate varicose veins. They are losing weight, exercise, wear compression stockings, elevate legs, and keep moving.

Ways to manage your weight. The first thing to do is drink plenty of water to help lose weight. Second, stay consistent in do not over eat. Third, be sure to get plenty of sleep, about seven to nine hours. Last, log-on to a weight-management website to help keep pounds off! Healthy eating! The five ways to a healthier life are: walk daily, socialize often, exercise regularly, try new things, and eat well. Be sure to eat five servings of fruits and veggies daily, use canola and olive oil when cooking, and eat whole grains, oats, rye grains, and unsalted nuts. Not sure what to order from a menu? Here are a few ways to stay away from fatty foods. They are house salad, no condiments, beware of cooking styles like no glazed, crispy, and crusted. What to order instead? The meats to order are steak that are sirloin, tenderloin, bottom, or top round and bone-in chicken dish. Tap away hunger for junk food by gently tap wrist, eyebrow, chin, and collarbone.

What to use for sinus pain? Inhale peppermint tea's vapor. Prevent heart disease by taking 360 mg Vitamin C and drink three glasses of cranberry juice. Stressed? Drink lemon balm tea. Taking B-complex reduces migraine pain. Flaxseed is good for menstrual cramps. Put flaxseed over yogurt, salads, and cereals.

8 EAT FIVE A DAY

FOR BREAKFAST

(1 each day)

1. Oatmeal with raisin and cinnamon along with fat-free milk.

2. Two whole-wheat waffles with peanut butter and one banana.

3. One or two eggs, (scrambled, poached, or hard boiled) with veggies along with one or two slices of whole-wheat toast with fruit jam and calcium-orange juice.

4. High fiber cereal with fruit and fat-free milk.

LUNCH

(1 each day)

1. One peanut butter and jelly sandwich on whole-wheat bread with baby carrots.

2. One tuna fish salad sandwich on whole-wheat bread with one slice low-fat cheese and baby spinach or romaine lettuce along with tomatoes and cucumbers.

3. One turkey sandwich on whole-wheat bread with one slice low-fat cheese and baby spinach or romaine lettuce along with tomatoes and cucumber and pistachios.

4. Egg salad sandwich on whole-wheat bread with slice low-fat cheese and baby spinach or romaine lettuce along with tomatoes and cucumbers.

5. One cup reduced-sodium soup, two slices of whole-wheat toast with one slice of fat-free

cheese along with tomatoes and baby carrots.

Dinner

(1 each day)

1. One grilled turkey patty on whole-wheat roll along with vegetables.

2. One grilled skinless barbecue chicken breast with Asian-style vegetables.

3. One grilled fish with lemon juice along with peas and carrots.

4. Small serving of brown rice with low-sodium chicken soup and vegetables.

5. Small serving of sweet potatoes and lots of vegetables.

6. Spinach and Romaine Salad with Strawberries and cooked cut-up chicken.

SNACKS

(2 each day)

1. One slice low-fat cheese with an apple.

2. One or two light non-fat yogurt with fruit.

3. One or two slices whole-wheat bread with peanut butter and one banana.

4. One 100 or fewer calorie snack.

5. One small pkg. raisins with one small pkg. of no salt nuts.

6. Cherry tomatoes, raw green beans, baby carrots, cucumbers, and sugar snap peas.

MAKE YOUR OWN MEALS

1. Use small portions of wheat pasta like spaghetti with lots of vegetables or green beans.

2. Eat small portions of meat with lots of vegetables.

3. Make your own vegetable salads with low-fat meats (cooked).

Please Note:

Wheat pasta, brown rice, corn, and sweet potatoes are starch that cannot be served with meat due to weight gain. Eat in moderation.

9 EXERCISES

Exercising can hurt if starting out at a fast pace. CDC (2003) stated, Use a sensible approach by starting out slowly and, begin by choosing moderate-intensity activities you enjoy the most (para 6)." There are many different kinds of exercise that a person can do, to lose weight and create energy. Some of them are yoga, aerobics, and weight for strength, exercise machines, stretches, running, dancing, swimming, pole exercising, boot camp, and ballet. Doing stretches before and after any exercise is an exceptional way of taking care of the body. For an exceptional set of exercise, all a person need is a weight bench, a few sets of dumbbells, and a stability ball. The entire time to do the exercises are 30-45 minutes for either the upper body or the lower body swimming, biking, jogging, walking on separate days, The weights are more effective than machines, improves balance, and coordination. When exercising standing up is to burn more calories, keep workout balanced, exercise all muscles equally, and sharing the time with a friend or a group club. The fitness clubs are a good way to get the exercise needed from aerobics to exercise machines. There are many of aerobics exercise tapes to buy in the store like dancing to the oldies, boot camp, and kickboxing that are fun to do, The way to reduce cellulites that are on the legs is to do the right type of exercises and do a 20-minute workout, three days a week.

Dancing is an exceptional way to get good exercise by helping to strengthen the whole body and reduce stress. To reduce stress is by remembering the dance steps and; it builds confidence. There are many types of dancing like square dancing, line dancing, ballroom, belly dancing, jazz, tap, modern, clogging, and ballet. The senior citizens like to go swimming to socialize and athletes do their training by swimming. Peterson (1996) stated, "Aquacise (water exercise) and many other types of recreational swimming are showing growing numbers of senior participants". Additionally, swimming is good for people who have health problems, have fun, or want to lose weight. When people go swimming at a gym that has a pool or at their home; they can do some exercising by running, walking, aerobics, kickboxing, yoga, or do a 30-minute workout. There many items to use when going to the pool like toys, dumbbells, paddles, beach balls, buoyancy belts, and kickboards. While swimming, it is very relaxing so much so; that it helps the whole body and reduces stress. Here is another way to lose weight and; it is pole dancing. Pole dancing was shone on one of the television shows that have been around for about two years. There are studios that have pole dancing in parts of the country and take a 50-minute session. Additionally, anyone can buy a portable exercise dance pole called Xpole online. Another exceptional cardio workout to use is The Body Burner and;

it looks like a small trampoline that comes with a training DVD. The Body Burner helps a person to lose weight, improves sports performance, and balance.

Now doctors say that the best exercise is walking every day as it controls weight, reduce body fat, reduce stress, lowers blood pressure, and reduces cholesterol, colon cancer, and stroke as well as less osteoarthritis pain with more flexibility. Many of the people use food for eating when they are stressed and when this happens; they gain weight, The best thing to do to help stop the eating binges is start writing a food journal by what was eaten and reason.

10 CONCLUSION

There are people out there that do not know how to lose weight properly, because the only way to lose weight is by eating healthy food and exercise on a daily basis. Some people go to a nutrition company, because; they believe that this is the only way to lose weight only to find that it did not work well as they did not add exercise to their diet. Since the people did not add exercise with their diet; they did not lose the weight and dropped out of the program. This shows that the only way to lose weight is by eating a healthy diet by cooking from scratch and exercise every day.

References

Anisman-Reiner, V (Sept 2, 2006) *Sugars: The Good*,

naturalmedicine.101.com,

http://naturalmedicine.suite101.com/article.cfm/sugars.

the.good

Anisman-Reiner, V (Sept, 9, 2006), *Sugars: The Bad*,

naturalmedicine.suie101.com,

http://naturalmedicine.suite101.com/article.cfm/sugars.

the.bad

Disease control and Prevention (CDC), (2/6, 2003), *Making*

Physical Activity Part of Your Life, WebMD,

http://www.webmd.com/fitness-exercise/physical-

activity-motivation

Harvard Health Publications, (April 2006), *Keeping*

Weight-loss Drugs in Perspective,

http://health.msn.com/dietfitness/articlepage.aspx?cp-

documentid=100134888

Cleveland Clinic, (2/2002), *Herbal Supplements: Helpful or Harmful?* Leonard, M. Pharm. D., http://www.clevelandclinic.org/heartcenter/pub/guide/prevention/alternative/herbals_theheart.htm

Internal Health Library, (November 30, 2006), *Therapies Juice Therapy*, Google, com, http://www.internalhealthlibrary.com/therapies/juice-therapy.htm

Peterson, C. A., (July 1996), *Aquatic Programming for Seniors*, National Recreation and Parks Association 1996, Gale Group 2004, http://findarticles.com/p/articles/mi.m1145/is.n7.v31/ai.18531674

Warner, J., (3/2, *2004), Have We Gone Carb Crazy?* WebMD, http://www.webmd.com/a-to-z-guides/features/low-carb-craze

ABOUT THE AUTHOR

While going to college, Elizabeth Carrell had done some research on health and nutrition for an essay. She discovered that many of the people are obese that she wanted to share all that she has learned today. Some of her new research is reading up on health magazines to find out the latest ways in helping oneself to lose weight and staying healthy. Some of her questions are: What does vinegar do for us? In what ways can a person keep from getting Alzheimer's disease? In what ways can a person lose weight and keep it off for good?